MIGHT *as* WELL *Laugh*

EMBRACING HUMOR IN DEMENTIA CARE

CONNIE ZENO

Copyright © 2024 Connie Zeno.

All rights reserved. No part of this book may be reproduced, stored, or transmitted by any means—whether auditory, graphic, mechanical, or electronic—without written permission of both publisher and author, except in the case of brief excerpts used in critical articles and reviews. Unauthorized reproduction of any part of this work is illegal and is punishable by law.

ISBN: 979-8-89419-152-2 (sc)
ISBN: 979-8-89419-153-9 (hc)
ISBN: 979-8-89419-154-6 (e)

Because of the dynamic nature of the Internet, any web addresses or links contained in this book may have changed since publication and may no longer be valid. The views expressed in this work are solely those of the author and do not necessarily reflect the views of the publisher, and the publisher hereby disclaims any responsibility for them.

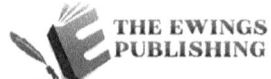

One Galleria Blvd., Suite 1900, Metairie, LA 70001
(504) 702-6708

The adage it takes a village to raise a child, well I submit to you that it takes a village to care for loved ones with dementia and physical disabilities. The care of family members with either physical or mental disabilities necessitates help from many sources.

I want to express my gratitude to our caregivers for all you did for Mom. The love and patience you displayed towards her has not gone unnoticed. I know my mother felt loved by you! Your selfless acts of kindness and generosity were over the top. I dedicate this book to you!

> *Thank you, Jackie Marcano.*
> *Thank you, Robin Lowe.*
> *Thank you, Carla Terrell.*

CONTENTS

Introduction. 1

Chapter 1:   My Story 5

Chapter 2:   Information. 9

Chapter 3:   My Purse was Stolen. 41

Chapter 4:   Help! 61

Chapter 5:   Going Home. 67

Notes 73

INTRODUCTION

Who said things are going to get better as we get older? Whoever said it has not experienced the getting older part of life.

I remember as a young girl sitting on the steps in front of my house with friends, daydreaming about what life would be like when we are all grown up. We expressed our dreams of being doctors, lawyers, firefighters, and astronauts with our goals of saving the world from diseases and traveling to star systems beyond our solar system. We would have four or five children and live happily ever after with our spouses, and of course, making a boatload of money was in the picture too. With our money, we would buy our parents new homes, and they would not have to work two or three jobs anymore to support their families. Those were going to be the days, to borrow a phrase, of "wine and roses."

Life has a way of coming at you fast with a reality check in hand. Gone are the dreamy-eyed days of make-believe. So here we are now some fifty or more years in the present.

Those dreams have evaporated long ago for most of us, and for others, some have realized them but not to the extent of their dreams. For many of us, we've had to settle for something less than what we hoped for on those hot summer days so long ago.

As I look back over my life, there are but a couple of things I would change; but otherwise, for me it has been a wonderful life. In all our daydreaming, it never occurred to any of us that one day we would be in a position of caring for our aging parents. That caring for them will come at the prime of our lives, when we are looking forward to retirement. Our preparation for the last thirty to forty years has been for that eventual day when we would call it quits, have that luncheon then go vacationing until we drop and, yes, spending time with the grands. Our thoughts regarding parents were they would at some point go into a retirement facility or they might remain in their home until the good Lord calls them home. They would still be able to care for themselves but just at a slower pace. Those of my generation never dreamed that we would be instrumental in caring for them and, in many cases, bringing them into our homes to live.

This book is in part informative, humorous, insightful and encouraging for all those experiencing caring for Mom, Dad or a family member. I hope you will find comfort in what is shared and knowing that it is our duty to care for our mothers and fathers. They have laid down their lives to care for us as we grew to maturity, so now it's our turn to honor them in their twilight years.

Might As Well Laugh will help you navigate times of frustration and will help keep your blood pressure at a reasonable level. Might as well laugh—what else are you going to do?

CHAPTER 1

My Story

*My son do not forget my law, but let your heart keep
my commands; For length of days and long life
and peace they will add to you.
Proverbs 3:1-2*

My story is typical of a young Black family trying to make it in the 1950s. Our household was a single-parent home. My family consisted of my mom, my brother, Keith, and myself. Our mother was breadwinner, father, mother, disciplinarian, and educator. Mom ran a tight ship. Her words were law, and we knew it. When we broke the rules, punishment was not far behind and that is exactly where it landed too! Mom loved God and she made sure we attended church on Sundays even when she was not feeling well. Mother suffered from chronic asthma.

She had to be very sick for us not to attend church, and the same goes for work. As a single parent, she could not afford to miss a day's work because there was no other money coming into our home. Many times, we witnessed Mom barely walking because of asthma. There were many days when Mom could not make it home because she was in the ER. She was such a regular patient that when she was brought in, the nurses directed the attendants to her familiar location. Mother chose to work the graveyard shift at the main Post Office on 30th Street in Philadelphia. By doing so, she got the night differential pay which we needed. I applaud Mom for keeping first things first.

What I mean by that is our mother's priority was taking care of her children, ensuring there was enough food in the house, paying the rent, utilities, providing clothes for her growing family and ensuring we have structure in our lives. Mom modeled before us a determination, tenacity, responsibility and a love for God that still, to this day, is embedded in Keith and me—unlike today's culture, where many single women with children are more concerned about having a boyfriend than caring for their children. Their children are left with unsavory men, and in some cases, they are abusing the children. Children are supposed to be safe within the home. The home is supposed to be a place of love, security and care given by parents or a parent. The home is supposed to be a sanctuary for them and not a den of terror and abuse. We never had to worry about this issue. Mom was zealous when it came to protecting her babies. And I am most appreciative to her that I did not have to be concerned about any man hurting me. Mother was the epitome of a "momma bear" protecting her young. For that, I am grateful to her.

Mother did not talk much about our father. However, it took her years to reveal what I now know about their relationship. We later discovered our father was mean, abusive, an alcoholic and a womanizer. Abusive to Mom but not towards us. I don't doubt some of the abuse was about us, but Mom took the direct hits, if you know what I mean. I believe the tremendous stress she was under opened the door to asthma and all the other underlying physical problems she had. When she got anxious, worried, and stressed, the asthma would flare up.

It was not easy in the 1950s for a single, attractive Black woman to make decent money. She faced prejudice, sexism, chauvinism, and bigotry but she did not allow it to deter her from her purpose. She was like the momma lion, knowing and doing what needed to be done because her pups depended on her for survival. We had extended family support that helped Mom in so many countless ways. They assisted by bringing us into their homes for the weekend so that Mother could rest and, in some cases, feel better. That was a blessing for us because it allowed Keith and me to spend time with our cousins. Thank God for family.

That was a brief glimpse into my family history which provides the backdrop for what this book is about. Knowing Mom, how she was back then (a no-nonsense "I will do it myself" kind of woman) to where we are today (a frail, forgetful, sometimes confused and sometimes angry nonagenarian) has been challenging, especially seeing her in this state. (Nonagenarian is 90 years old and above.)

The title of this book was given to me by my husband, Henderson Zeno. I was telling him one day of a frustrating experience with Mom and his reply to me was "You might as well laugh, because anything else will cause your blood pressure to rise." He was so right. So, why was I allowing my mom or the situation to cause my blood pressure to rise? Partly because I did not know how to handle situations with Mom. At the end of the day, it was not worth getting my blood pressure to rise over nonsensical stuff. God even says in His Word, *"A merry heart does good like medicine" (Proverbs 17:22).*

There are just some things you might as well laugh about. So here is our story—our journey with Mom through dementia.

CHAPTER 2

Information

"My people are destroyed for a lack of knowledge / understanding"
Hosea 4:6

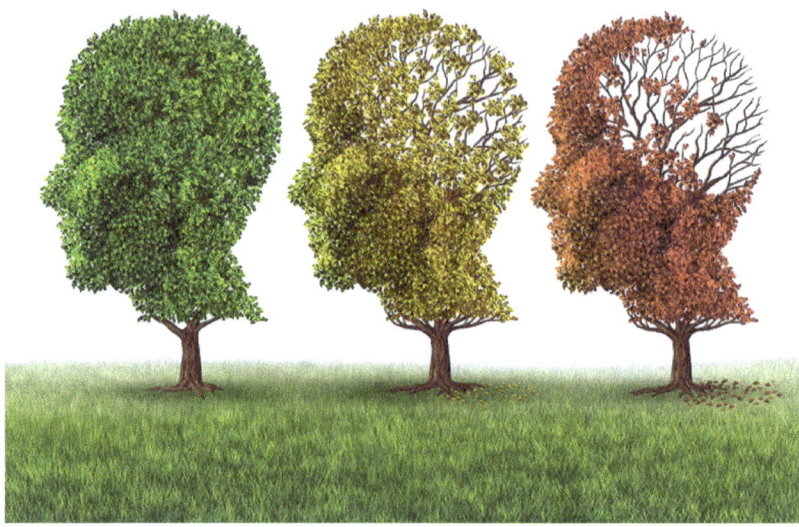

A group of trees, representing the human brain, transitions through the colors of autumn, shedding leaves that symbolize diminishing intelligence. Against a white backdrop, the image portrays the gradual loss of memory and brain aging due to dementia and Alzheimer's disease.

This picture gives a vivid visual of how the brain looks as dementia progresses. As the onset of dementia increases, more leaves fade away from the branches until it looks like barren branches. This directly correlates to the decline in memory, speech, and reasoning abilities, reflecting the onset of diminished cognitive capacity within the brain. Memory, speech, and reasoning aren't the sole casualties of dementia. Emotions and physical abilities are affected too.

This journey with God and Mom has made me realize just how ignorant I was regarding dementia. In my lack of understanding to what happens to the brain experiencing signs of dementia, I thought it was a matter of taking some over-the-counter meds to help boost memory or one needed to engage in brain exercises, helping the brain to remember. Rather, it is much more complex than I initially thought. So, for the next few pages, we will look at some scientific data and evidence regarding the brain, memory, and the progression of the disease.

Disclaimer: I am not a doctor or scientist. The information used are from creditable doctors and organizations.

What is dementia? And how is it different from Alzheimer's disease?

Dementia and Alzheimer's disease aren't the same. Dementia is an overall term used to describe symptoms that impact memory, performance of daily activities and communication abilities. Alzheimer's is the most common type of dementia. Alzheimer's disease gets worse with time and affects memory, language and thoughts.

While younger people can develop dementia or Alzheimer's disease, your risk increases as you age. Still, neither is considered a normal part of aging.

Although symptoms of the two conditions may overlap, distinguishing them is important for management and treatment.

The information below is cited from WebMD LLC 2020.

Dementia is a syndrome, not a disease. A syndrome is a group of symptoms that doesn't have a definitive diagnosis. Dementia is an umbrella term that Alzheimer's disease can fall under. It can occur due to a variety of conditions, the most common of which is Alzheimer's disease.

Dementia is the name for a group of brain disorders that make it hard to remember, think clearly, make decisions, or even control your emotions. Alzheimer's disease is one of those disorders, but there are many different types and causes of dementia. To maintain the focus of this book, I will not delve into all the different diseases caused by dementia. I am only giving a broad-level view of this syndrome and how it has manifested in my mother's life.

Dementia isn't just about simple memory mishaps—like forgetting someone's name or where you parked. A person with dementia has a hard time with at least two of the following:

- Memory
- Communication and speech
- Focus and concentration

- Reasoning and judgment
- Visual perception (can't see the difference in colors or detect movement or sees things that aren't there)

Since some types of dementia share similar symptoms, it can be hard for a doctor to figure out which one you or your loved one has. Be sure to tell him about all symptoms, medications and alcohol use, and previous illnesses to help him make the right diagnosis.

Alzheimer's Disease (AD)

This is the most common type of dementia. About 60% to 80% of people who have dementia have Alzheimer's. It's a progressive condition, which means it gets worse over time, and it usually affects people over 65 years old. There's currently no cure.

It happens when proteins (called plaques) and fibers (called tangles) build up in your brain and block nerve signals and destroy nerve cells. Memory loss may be mild at first, but symptoms become worse over time.

It gets more difficult to carry on a conversation or perform everyday tasks. Confusion, aggression, and mood changes are other common symptoms.

A doctor can't say you have Alzheimer's with absolute certainty, but there are things he can do to be fairly sure.

They include tests of your attention, memory, language and vision, and looking at images of the brain. These images are taken with an MRI (magnetic resonance imaging), which uses powerful magnets and radio waves to make detailed pictures.

Damage to the brain begins years before symptoms appear. Abnormal protein deposits form plaques and tangles in the brain of someone with Alzheimer's disease. Connections between cells are lost, and they begin to die. In advanced cases, the brain shows significant shrinkage.

It's impossible to diagnose Alzheimer's with complete accuracy while a person is alive. The diagnosis can only be confirmed when the brain is examined under a microscope during an autopsy. However, specialists are able to make the correct diagnosis up to 90 percent of the time.

Other Types of Dementia:

Vascular dementia: This is the second most common type. About 1 in 10 people who have dementia have vascular dementia, which happens when there's not enough blood going to your brain. This can be caused by damage to your blood vessels or blockages that lead to mini-strokes or brain bleeding. Doctors used to call it multi-infarct or post-stroke dementia.

Unlike Alzheimer's disease, memory loss isn't the typical first symptom. Instead, people with vascular dementia can have different signs, depending on the area of the brain that's affected, such as problems with planning or judgment. No drugs have been approved to treat this type of dementia, but you can do some things to keep your brain and blood vessels healthy and try to prevent future damage. These include exercising, eating well, and not smoking.

Dementia with Lewy bodies: Lewy bodies are abnormal clumps of a protein called alpha-synuclein. They build up in your cortex, the part of your brain that handles learning and memory.

This type of dementia causes problems with attention and things like driving early on, along with sleeping issues, seeing things that aren't there (hallucinations), and slowed, unbalanced movements, similar to Parkinson's disease symptoms. Memory loss tends to show up later in the disease.

Mixed dementia: Sometimes, a person has brain changes caused by more than one type of dementia. This is called mixed dementia. For example, you may have blocked or damaged blood vessels in your brain (vascular dementia) and brain plaques and tangles (Alzheimer's disease) at the same time.

Frontotemporal dementia: This form of dementia involves the loss of nerve cells in the front and side areas of your brain—behind your forehead and ears. Personality and behavior changes and trouble with language are the main symptoms. Some people also have a hard time with writing and comprehension.

Symptoms usually show up around age 60—earlier than they usually start with Alzheimer's disease. Types of frontotemporal dementia include behavioral variant FTD (bvFTD), primary progressive aphasia, Pick's disease, corticobasal degeneration, and progressive supranuclear palsy.

Creutzfeldt-Jakob Disease (CJD): This rare form of dementia happens when a protein, called a prion, folds into an abnormal shape, and other prions start to do the same. This damages brain cells and triggers a fast mental decline.

People with CJD also have mood changes, confusion, twitchy or jerky movements, and trouble walking. Sometimes, the disease is passed down through families, but it also can happen for no known reason.

Symptoms of dementia

It's easy to overlook the early symptoms of dementia, which can be mild. It often begins with simple episodes of forgetfulness. People with dementia have trouble keeping track of time and tend to lose their way in familiar settings.

As dementia progresses, forgetfulness and confusion grow. It becomes harder to recall names and faces. Personal care becomes a problem. Obvious signs of dementia include repetitious questioning, inadequate hygiene, and poor decision-making.

In the most advanced stage, people with dementia become unable to care for themselves. They will struggle even more with keeping track of time and remembering people and places they are familiar with. Behavior continues to change and can turn into depression and aggression.

(cited from WebMD LLC 2020)

I will be mentioning the highly noteworthy seven stages of Alzheimer's, also known as the Global Deterioration Scale (GDS), which were developed by Dr. Barry Reisberg, Director of the Fisher Alzheimer's Disease Education and Research program at NYU Grossman School of Medicine. This comprehensive guideline, cited from www.alzinfo.org, is widely used by professionals and caregivers globally to accurately identify and understand the progression of Alzheimer's disease in patients.

STAGE 1: NO DEMENTIA SEEN

At any age, persons may be free of objective or subjective symptoms of cognitive and functional decline, as well as of associated behavioral and mood changes. We call these mentally healthy persons at any age, stage 1, or normal.

STAGE 2: SUBJECTIVE MEMORY LOSS

Many people over the age of 65 complain of cognitive and/or functional difficulties. Elderly persons with these symptoms report that they can no longer remember names as easily as they could 5 or 10 years previously; they can also have trouble recalling where they have recently placed things.

Various terms have been suggested for this condition, but subjective cognitive decline is presently the widely accepted terminology. These symptoms by definition, are not notable to intimates or other external observers of the person with subjective cognitive decline. Persons with these symptoms decline at higher rates than similarly aged persons and similarly healthy persons who are free of subjective complaints. Research has shown that this stage of subjective cognitive decline lasts 15 years in otherwise healthy persons.

STAGE 3: MILD COGNITIVE IMPAIRMENT

Persons at this stage manifest deficits which are subtle, but which are noted by persons who are closely associated with the person with mild cognitive impairment. The subtle deficits may become manifest in diverse ways. For example, a person with mild cognitive impairment (MCI) may noticeably repeat queries. The capacity to perform executive functions also becomes compromised. Commonly, for persons who are still working in complex occupational settings, job performance may decline. For those required to master new job skills, such as a computer or other machinery, decrements in these capacities may become evident.

MCI persons who are not employed, but who plan complex social events, such as dinner parties, may manifest declines in their ability to organize such events. This may be an early stage of Alzheimer's, however, it is important for the person to seek medical help as soon as possible, to determine if a broad variety of medical conditions may be causing or contributing to the person's difficulties. Blood tests and an MRI of the brain should be obtained to assist in determining if the individual has MCI due to Alzheimer's and whether there are other causes or contributing conditions to the person's cognitive decline.

Some MCI persons may manifest concentration deficits. Many persons with these symptoms begin to experience anxiety, which may be overtly evident.

The prognosis for persons with these subtle symptoms of impairment is variable. The average total duration of the MCI stage in otherwise healthy persons is seven years. In persons who are not called upon to perform complex, occupational and or social tasks, symptoms in this MCI stage may not become evident to family members or friends until midway or near the end of this stage.

Management of persons in this stage includes counseling regarding the desirability of continuing in a complex and demanding occupational role. Sometimes, a "strategic withdrawal" in the form of retirement, may alleviate psychological stress and reduce both personal and overtly manifest anxiety.

STAGE 4: MODERATE COGNITIVE DECLINE (MILD DEMENTIA)

The diagnosis of Alzheimer's disease can be made with considerable accuracy in this stage. The most common functioning deficit in these persons is a decreased ability to manage instrumental (complex) activities of daily life, which may hinder their ability to live independently. For the stage 4 person, this may become evident in the form of difficulties in paying rent and other bills, not being able to write out checks with the correct date or amount without assistance; the inability to market for personal items and groceries or order from a menu in a restaurant. Persons who previously prepared meals for family members and/or guests begin to manifest decreased performance in these skills.

Symptoms of memory loss also become evident in this stage. For example, seemingly major recent events, such as a holiday or visit with a relative may not be remembered. Obvious mistakes in remembering the day of the week, month or season of the year may occur.

Persons at this stage can still generally recall their correct current address; they can usually correctly remember the weather conditions outside. Significant current events, including the name of a prominent head of state, will likely be recalled easily. Despite the obvious deficits in cognition, persons at this stage can still potentially survive independently in community settings.

The dominant mood at this stage is frequently what psychiatrists term a flattening of affect and withdrawal. In other words, the person with mild Alzheimer's disease often seems less emotionally responsive than previously. This absence of emotional responsivity is related to the person's denial of their deficit, which is often also notable at this stage. Although the person is aware of their shortcomings, this awareness of decreased intellectual capacity is painful for them. Hence, the psychological defense mechanism known as denial, whereby the person with Alzheimer's disease seeks to hide their deficit, even from themselves, becomes operative. Also, the person withdraws from participation in activities such as conversations.

In the absence of complicating medical pathology, the diagnosis of Alzheimer's disease (AD) can be made with considerable certainty from the beginning of this stage. Studies indicate that the duration of this stage of mild AD has a mean of approximately two years in otherwise healthy persons.

STAGE 5: MODERATELY SEVERE COGNITIVE DECLINE (MODERATE DEMENTIA)

In this stage, deficits are of sufficient magnitude as to prevent catastrophe-free, independent community survival. The characteristic functional change in this stage is early deficits in basic activities of daily life. This is manifest in a decrement in the ability to choose the proper clothing to wear for the weather conditions or for everyday circumstances. Some persons with Alzheimer's disease begin to wear the same clothing day after day unless reminded to change. The mean duration of this stage is 1.5 years.

The person with Alzheimer's disease can no longer manage on their own. There is generally someone who is assisting in providing adequate and proper food, as well as assuring that the rent and utilities are paid and the finances are taken care of. For those who are not properly supervised, predatory strangers may become a problem. Very common reactions for persons at this stage who are not given adequate support are behavioral problems such as anger and suspiciousness.

Cognitively, persons at this stage frequently cannot recall major events and aspects of their current life such as the name of the current head of state, the weather conditions of the day, or their correct current address. Characteristically, some of these important aspects of current life are recalled, but not others. Also, the information is loosely held, so, for example, the person with moderate Alzheimer's disease may recall their correct address on certain occasions, but not others.

Remote memory also suffers to the extent that persons may not recall the names of some of the schools which they attended for many years, and from which they graduated. Orientation may be compromised to the extent that the correct year may not be recalled. Calculation deficits may be of such magnitude that an educated person has difficulty correctly counting backward from 20 by 2s.

Functionally, persons at this stage commonly have incipient difficulties with basic activities of daily life. The characteristic deficit of this type is decreased ability to independently choose proper clothing to wear, in accordance with the weather conditions and the events of the day. In otherwise healthy persons this stage lasts an average of approximately 1.5 years.

STAGE 6: SEVERE COGNITIVE DECLINE (MODERATELY SEVERE DEMENTIA)

Stage 6a

At this stage, the ability to perform basic activities of daily life becomes compromised. Functionally, five successive substages are identifiable. Persons initially in stage 6a, in addition to having lost the ability to choose their clothing without assistance, begin to require assistance in putting on their clothing properly. Unless supervised, the person with Alzheimer's disease may put their clothing on backward, they may have difficulty putting their arm in the correct sleeve, or they may dress in the wrong sequence.

The total duration of the stage of moderately severe Alzheimer's disease (stage 6a through 6e) is approximately 2.5 years in otherwise healthy persons.

Stage 6b

At approximately the same point in the evolution of AD, but generally just a little later in the temporal sequence, AD persons lose the ability to bathe without assistance (stage 6b). Characteristically, the earliest and most common deficit in bathing is difficulty adjusting the temperature of the bath water. Once the caregiver adjusts the temperature of the bath water, the AD person can still potentially otherwise bathe independently. As this stage evolves, additional deficits occur in bathing and dressing independently. In this 6b substage, AD persons generally develop deficits in other modalities of daily hygiene such as properly brushing their teeth.

Stages 6c, 6d, 6e

With the further evolution of AD, persons lose the ability to manage independently the mechanics of toileting (stage 6c). Unless supervised, the person with AD may place the toilet tissue in the wrong place. The AD person may also forget to flush the toilet properly. As the disease evolves in this stage, AD person subsequently become incontinent. Generally, urinary incontinence occurs first (stage 6d), then fecal incontinence occurs (stage 6e). The incontinence can be treated, or even initially prevented entirely in many cases, by frequent toileting. Subsequently, strategies for managing incontinence, including appropriate bedding, absorbent undergarments, etc., become necessary.

In this sixth stage cognitive deficits are generally so severe that persons will display little or no knowledge when queried regarding such major aspects of their current life circumstances as their current address or the weather conditions of the day.

In this stage, the AD person's cognitive deficits are generally of such magnitude that the person with AD may, at times, confuse their wife with their mother or otherwise misidentify or be uncertain of the identity of close family members. At the end of this sixth stage, the ability to speak begins to break down.

Recall of current events in this 6th moderately severe stage of AD is generally deficient to the extent that the AD person frequently cannot name the current national head of state or other, similarly prominent newsworthy figures. Persons at this sixth stage will most often not be able to recall the names of any of the schools which they attended. They may or may not recall such basic life events as the names of their parents, their former occupation or the country in which they were born. They still have some knowledge of their own names; however, persons in this stage may mistake the identity of persons, even close family members. Calculation ability is frequently so severely compromised at this stage that even well-educated persons with AD have difficulty counting backward consecutively from 10 by 1s.

Emotional changes generally become most overt and disturbing in this sixth stage of AD. Although these emotional changes may, in part, have a neurochemical basis, they are also clearly related to the AD person's psychological reaction to their circumstances. For example, because of their cognitive deficits, persons at this stage can no longer channel their energies into productive activities. Consequently, persons may begin to fidget, to pace, to move objects around, or to manifest other forms of purposeless or inappropriate activities. Because of their fear, frustration and shame regarding their circumstances, these persons frequently develop verbal outbursts and also threatening, even violent behavior. Because these AD persons can no longer survive independently, they commonly develop a fear of being left alone. Treatment of these and other behavioral and psychological symptoms involves counseling regarding appropriate activities and the psychological impact of the illness on the person with AD frequently in combination with pharmacological interventions.

The mean duration of this sixth stage of AD is approximately 2.5 years. As this stage comes to an end, the AD person, who is doubly incontinent and needs assistance with dressing and bathing, begins to manifest overt breakdown in the ability to articulate sentences and words. Stuttering (verbigeration), neologisms, making up nonexistent words, and/or an increased paucity of speech, become manifest.

STAGE 7: VERY SEVERE COGNITIVE DECLINE (SEVERE DEMENTIA)

At this stage, AD persons require continuous assistance with basic activities of daily life for survival. Six consecutive functional substages can be identified over the course of this final seventh stage. Early in this stage, speech has become so circumscribed, as to be limited to approximately a half-dozen intelligible words or fewer (stage 7a). As this stage progresses, speech becomes even more limited to, at most, a single intelligible word (stage 7b). Once intelligible speech is lost, the ability to ambulate independently (without assistance), is invariably lost. However, ambulatory ability may be compromised at the end of the sixth stage and in the early portion of the seventh stage by concomitant physical disability, poor care, medication side-effects or other factors. Conversely, superb care provided in the early seventh stage, and particularly in stage 7b, can postpone the onset of loss of ambulation. However, under ordinary circumstances, stage 7a has a mean duration of approximately 1 year, and stage 7b has a mean duration of approximately 1.5 years.

In persons with AD who remain alive, stage 7c lasts approximately 1 year, after which persons with AD lose the ability not only to ambulate independently but also to sit up independently (stage 7d), At this point in the evolution, the person will fall over when seated unless there are armrests to assist in sitting up in the chair.

This 7d substage lasts approximately 1 year. AD persons who survive subsequently lose the ability to smile (stage 7e). At this substage only grimacing facial movements are observed in place of smiles. This 7e substage lasts a mean of approximately 1.5 years. It is followed in survivors by a final 7f substage, in which AD persons additionally lose the ability to hold up their head independently.

Persons can survive in this final 7f substage indefinitely; however, most persons with AD succumb at various points during the course of stage 7 to pneumonia, infected ulcerations, or other conditions.

With the advent of the seventh stage of AD, certain physical and neurological changes become increasingly evident. One of these changes is physical rigidity. Evident rigidity upon examination of the passive range of motion of major joints, such as the elbow, is present in the great majority of persons with AD throughout the course of the seventh stage.

In many persons with AD, this rigidity appears to be a precursor to the appearance of overt physical deformities in the form of contractures. Contractures are irreversible deformities which prevent the passive or active range of motion of joints. In the early seventh stage (7a and 7b), approximately 40% of AD persons manifest these deformities. Later in the seventh stage, in immobile persons with AD (from stage 7d to 7f), nearly all AD persons manifest contractures in multiple extremities and joints.

Neurological reflex changes also become evident in stage 7 AD persons. Particularly notable is the emergence of so-called 'infantile', 'primitive' or 'developmental' reflexes which are present in the infant but which disappear in the toddler. These reflexes, including the grasp reflex, the sucking reflex, and the Babinski plantar extensor reflex, are increasingly present as the stage 7 AD person's condition advances. Because of the greater physical size and strength of the AD person in comparison to an infant, these reflexes can be very strong and can impact both positively and negatively on the care provided to the person with AD. AD persons commonly die during the course of the seventh stage. The mean point of demise is when persons with AD lose the ability to ambulate and to sit up independently (stages 7c and 7d).

The most frequent proximate cause of death in persons with Alzheimer's is pneumonia. Aspiration is one common cause of terminal pneumonia. Another common cause of demise in AD is infected decubital ulcerations. AD persons in the seventh stage are also vulnerable to all of the common causes of mortality in the elderly including stroke, heart disease, and cancer. Some AD persons in this final stage appear to succumb to no identifiable condition other than AD.

(Cited from https://www.alzinfo.org/understand-alzheimers/clinical-stages-of-alzheimers/)

During my experience with Mother, she has exhibited memory loss, confusion, depression, aggression, loss of focus, difficulty communicating, and a decline in her reasoning and judgment. This has made it very challenging caring for her. I had to step back and realize the person I see now is not the same person who raised me. She is partially there, at best, but most times we are communicating with someone who is struggling within herself.

Our family is learning new ways of interacting and caring for Mom. There are days where the woman living with us doesn't know or recognize her family and days when it seems like we stepped back in time as far as our relationship goes like nothing has changed. Then there are days where she just cries and cries. I feel so helpless in these situations. And then there are days where she is angry at everyone. A sense of riding a rollercoaster seems to be our norm. The mood swings keep us on our toes. I cannot imagine what she is going through.

As I said in the first chapter, my mom was a very independent, strong, confident woman. As I look at her today, she bears little semblance to the person she once was. One might say, "Afterall, she is 91 years old. What do you expect?" I get it. But her sister, who is 94 years old, still possesses a fiery spirit and a tenacity that I marvel at. She still goes to work and drives her car. So, what happened in my mother's case? Why has her cognitive vitality been siphoned away? Where is the spitfire of a woman I've known all my life? Where did she go?

Let's look at the spiritual side of this. Mom attended church all her life. She was a member of North Penn Baptist Church, then a member of Triumph Baptist Church in Philadelphia, Pennsylvania. Just attending church does not make one spiritually strong. As believers, we are encouraged to not forsake the assembling together. Great! But we are also directed by the Lord Jesus to abide in His Word and allow His Word to abide in us.

"If you abide in My Word, you are My disciples indeed. And you shall know the truth and the truth shall make you free." John 8:31

"If you abide in Me and My words abide in you, you will ask what you desire, and it shall be done for you." John 15:7

"Your Word I have hidden in my heart, that I might not sin against You." Psalm 119:11

"I beseech you therefore, brethren by the mercies of God, that you present your bodies a living sacrifice, holy acceptable to God, which is your reasonable service.

And do not be conformed to this world, but be transformed by the renewing of your mind, that you may prove what is that good and acceptable and perfect will of God." Romans 12:1,2

It is scripturally clear that we are not to live by food alone but by every Word of God. Natural food feeds the physical body. God's Word feeds our spirit. Much too often, our physical bodies are better fed than our spirits. As born-again people, we are supposed to be sustained by God's Word. It is His Word that heals us, delivers us, renews our minds, and keeps us connected to our Father. It also cleanses us of the gunk and muck of the world. So, when it came to my mother, she did not have a revelation about God's Word being food for her soul. Therefore, God's Word was relegated to stories of the past. The Word as a vital necessity for living, like food for her body, was not a revelation in her life.

Sadly, many of God's people are not taught His Word. They are preached at, hyped up, and stirred up with music, and they leave church buildings every Sunday with nothing much to live on. Nothing of substance was spoken there, resulting in people leaving in the very same condition as when they entered. Lives were not impacted by God's Word. His Word, if taken as prescribed, will change you, heal you, deliver you, affirm your identity in Christ and much, much more. Many pastors will give an account to the Lord Jesus what they have fed the sheep. Woe to you, shepherds that care not for the sheep.

After His resurrection, the third time Jesus showed Himself to His disciples.

"So, when they had eaten breakfast, Jesus said to Simon Peter, 'Simon, son of Jonah do you love Me more than these?" He said to Him, "Yes, Lord; You know that I love You." He said to him, "<u>Feed</u> My lambs." He said to him a second time, "Simon, son of Jonah, do you love Me?" He said to Him, "Yes, Lord, You know that I love You." He said to him, "<u>Tend</u> My sheep." He said to him the third time, "Simon son of Jonah, do you love Me?" Peter was grieved because He said to Him the third time, "Do you love Me?" And he said to Him, Lord, You know all things; You know that I love You." Jesus said to him "<u>Feed</u> My sheep." John 21:15-17

Jesus gave Peter a charge. Regardless men, women, or children, they all need to be cared for and fed by the leadership of Christ's church among the nations. It was true then and it is true today.

This does not absolve us from digging into God's Word and believing His Word for ourselves. We are not created to be dependent on someone else doing our reading and praying and believing. We are created to have a personal relationship with our Lord. Pastors and leaders are given to help us in our journey. They should be pointing the way. We serve a personal God, so it is incumbent for each of us to study to show ourselves approved by God by allowing His Word to abide in us as we abide in His Word. That is a dual task—allowing the Word to live in us and we stay in the Word. The word *"abide"* means *to live in, to stay, remain, to be in a state that begins and continues, to follow Jesus' example of a life obedient to the will of God.*

There is so much that is competing for our time and attention that we must, on purpose, make time for God and His Word.

Romans 12: 2 says *"that we are to renew our minds with the Word of God."*

When we immerse ourselves in His Word, we become one with the Word. The Word of God has properties that can and will heal the mind. Why would the Lord require a renewed mind? When a person accepts Jesus as their Lord and Savior, their spirit is made new.

Therefore, if anyone is in Christ, he is a new creation; old things have passed away and behold, all things have become new.
2 Corinthians 5:17

The new birth experience occurs in the spirit of a man. This is where the reality of *"**all things have become new**"* happens. Yet, nothing was done with our soul or our physical body. The renewing of our soul is accomplished when we feed on God's Word. It is the result of washing and cleansing by His Word. It sets our thought patterns in order, heals our soul from emotional trauma and sickness, etc. We will begin to have new ways of thinking, new attitudes towards people, God, and circumstances.

> *"Stop imitating the ideals and opinions of the culture around you but be inwardly transformed by the Holy Spirit through **<u>a total reformation of how you think</u>**. This will empower you to discern God's will as you live a beautiful life, satisfying and perfect in His eyes. Romans 12:2 TPT*

The Lord insists on us having a total reformation of how we think. Reformation is a re-formatting of our thought processes. When we are born into this world, we are taught to think according to our ethic culture, family traditions, and the culture at large. Therefore, when we get saved by accepting Jesus Christ as our personal Lord and Savior, the Lord then requires us to think anew. This new way of thinking and living becomes a life-long process, a transformation within via the Word of God. When God called Abraham, He required him to leave his country, his family and everything that he was familiar with. Why? Because God had a plan for Abraham that would require a brand-new way of thinking and believing.

> *Now the Lord had said to Abram: "Get out of your country, from your family and from your father's house to a land that I will show you. I will make you a great nation; I will bless you and make your name great; and you shall be a blessing." Genesis 12:1-2*

God's plan for you and I are good, to give us a hope and a future, but we cannot advance into it without a renewed mind.

The mind is a leader or forerunner of all our actions. Our actions are a direct result of our thoughts. If we have negative thoughts, we will have negative results in life. If, on the other hand, our minds are being renewed with God's Word and by the Holy Spirit, we will experience the life that Jesus died for and gave to us. We are not to copy the behavior and customs of this world but let God transform us into a new person by changing the way we think. By doing so, we will learn to know God's will for us, which is good and pleasing and perfect.

His Word has a profound effect on our brain function. The brain and the mind are not synonymous. The brain is the physical organ, and the mind is the internal processes. For example, a computer: Just like the hard drive is the hardware for the computer, so is our brain for us. As the software is for the computer, so is our mind. We must constantly update the software of our minds. Our software must be re-formatted with God's Word.

In Dr. Caroline Leaf's book, **"Who Switched Off My Brain?"** she describes the anatomy of a thought. *She says,*

> *"Every thought whether it is positive or negative goes through the same cycle when it forms. Thoughts are basically electrical impulses, chemicals, and neurons. They look like trees with branches. As thoughts grow and become permanent, more branches grow, and the connections become stronger. As we change our thinking, some*

branches go away, new one's form, the strength of the connections change and the memories network with other thoughts. Thoughts are memories that are stored in the unconscious or subconscious mind."
(Cited from Who Switched Off My Brain?)

At one time, scientists promoted the hypothesis that once brain cells died, the body did not replace or generate new cells. However, this theory has been proven wrong. The brain has the capacity to generate new cells. New cells are formed when the brain is given new thoughts to process. You see, the brain establishes highways or patterns where our thoughts travel. As we age, if we continue thinking the way we have always thought, then the same patterns of thoughts develop grooves in the mind. For example, if you have a negative thought about a situation or an individual, all the emotions and chemicals associated with that thought flood your system, and you can feel like the event just happened because there have been well-established grooves related to this particular thought or event when you think of it.

'Thoughts are not only scientifically measurable, but we can verify how they affect our bodies. We can actually feel our thoughts through our emotions. Emotions are involved in every thought we build, ever have built and ever will build. In fact, for every memory you make, you have a corresponding emotion attached to it, which is stored in your brain and has a photocopy in your body's cells.' Who Switched Off My Brain?

When we think new thoughts, it forces the brain to make new patterns. In doing so, the brain must create new cells for the new thought highway or pattern. This is renewing the mind. Continuing to think the way we've always thought makes the grooves deeper. Over time, if the mind is not given new information and required to think differently, the thought highway gets clogged with plaque. The plaque builds up and causes disjointed speech, memory loss, and all the signs of dementia become evident. The plaque obstructs the electrical impulses, disrupting the normal thought pathway. Some of the suggested treatments for dementia patients is to stimulate other parts of the brain. Areas in the brain that are created through artistic expression is encouraged as well as the musical side. This gives the brain the opportunity to make new highways or patterns. Brain exercises are also encouraged to help the memory portion of the brain.

My mother, as stated earlier, lived under stress for most of my growing-up years. I believe the negative impact of stress, negative thoughts and an unrenewed mind contributed to the cause of dementia in her life. So here we are now, dealing with Mom and the effects of dementia. In this chapter, I just wanted to provide a surface view of dementia, its effects, and its effects on my mom, family, and friends. I hope this chapter has provided some insight into this malady. I would encourage you to get Dr. Leaf's book, "Who Switched Off My Brain?" The information contained in it has helped our family to understand the physiological workings of the brain.

The next chapter are selected humorous stories of Mom and friends who have walked through this process with loved ones.

CHAPTER 3

My Purse was Stolen

"For you shall go out with joy; and be led out with peace."
Isaiah 55:12

This is the chapter where we can laugh about some of the funniest and quirkiest things that we have witnessed and experienced. As I recall the events, I want you to understand that in no way am I making fun of my mother or anyone else, for that matter, but our stories are similar to others who are going through or have gone through the process with a loved one with dementia.

The early signs of something amiss with mom went unnoticed by me. In 2015, our conversation a few times revolved around her purse. She told me she was bringing groceries to the house and left her purse on the car seat and a couple boys stole her purse out of her car. She had the house and car keys in her hand, but all her identification was gone.

Another occasion, someone stole her purse from her house. She had no specifics about a break-in, only her purse was stolen. I advised her to contact the police department. She assured me she would do it, but she did not. We later learned the issue with her purse was in her mind. The purse was never lost but misplaced by her.

In 2016, she reported to me again her purse was stolen—this time from the supermarket. Later that year, I came home and discovered the supposedly stolen purse in her house. In questioning Mom, she could not tell me how or when the purse was returned. She had a specific black purse she used constantly. It was her favorite. I must say that purse has made more resurrections than Lazarus. It has made more comebacks than Michael Jordan. After talking with a few of Mom's friends, they told me her purse was never stolen. She misplaced it. I started noticing her memory recall was spotty, yet still I was not concerned, just chalked it up to getting old.

In 2017, my husband and I were flying into Philadelphia International. Arriving at 11:15 p.m. I would usually reserve a shuttle ride, but at my mother's insistence that she pick us up, I cancelled my reservations. We arrived on time. At midnight, I got a call from a security guard from a local college that my mother was there and she did not know how to get to the airport. The security guard eventually escorted Mom to the airport. On arrival, she was confused and nervous. It took us a bit to calm her down.

During our stay, I began to see more things out of order in her home, especially her bill paying. Most of her bills were two or three months late. I found checks written for particular bills with a statement of *"sorry for being late but my purse was stolen."* It was then I decided to assume the responsibility of paying her bills. This was done with her permission, of course. I think it came as a relief for her too.

We also noticed things were not operating in the house like the TV, computers, lamps, and internet. This was because she was unplugging everything except the phone. This was true every time we came for a visit.

From this point forward, we took a proactive role in Mom's affairs. This was very time-consuming because her bookkeeping skills were all over the place; and when I say all over the place, I mean all over the place. There was no order to how she paid her bills, nor did we know who she owed. Mind you, Mom has always been conscientious about paying her bills and paying them on time! I remember countless lectures from her regarding this matter. It took a couple of trips back to Philly to round up all her debt and contact her debtors to sort things out. Many of her creditors were understanding and were willing to work with me.

In the middle of all this, Mom would accuse me of taking her money and not being a good daughter to her. I showed her the ledger of her finances and where she was currently in respect to her debt, but that was not enough for her. She, to this day, accuses me of spending her money with claims she has nothing.

I came to the realization just how out of touch with reality she had become. This is an indicator of the disease progression. I had to keep this in mind when dealing with Mom. At times I would revert in my mind, thinking she is the person I've known before the dementia. When this happened, it presented a challenge in my relationship with her. I'll talk more about this in the next chapter.

In 2017, we began the process of looking for a place for Mom. Our plan was to place her in a facility in Philadelphia because it was close to her church and some family members. We gathered moving boxes for Mom to pack up her things. We returned to Philly on two separate occasions only to find the moving boxes empty and in the same place where we left them. Mom would tell us that she was trying to pack but the job seemed so big. Then we would pack things, and she would remove them from the boxes. Keith, my brother, finally had to give her a project in a different part of the house. That kept her busy for a hot minute.

By the end of that year, we were all set to move her into the assisted living facility when she took a negative turn in her cognitive abilities. This caused the monthly care cost to increase because now she needed memory care. The cost exceeded her monthly annuity and social security. So, <u>now</u> we <u>must</u> sell her home prior to her going into a home. We felt the urgency of the moment, but unfortunately Mom did not share the same urgency. She kept telling us she could take care of herself and stay in her home and she was just fine on her own, but the reality of the situation said something totally different. Trying to convince her of that was a monumental task. The more we tried convincing her that she could not live alone any longer, the more she dug her heels in that she could live independently. Our trips home were short stays because we still had jobs and families to go home to. So we left with the situation unresolved.

Enter 2018, an interesting year, to say the least. Throughout the year, we received calls from well-meaning people who were concerned about Mom's welfare. She wasn't eating well, some said. She was confused others said. There were concerns about her driving especially at night, concerns about her cooking and leaving the gas on, concerns about her being alone in the house, etc.

I returned home in the spring of 2018. There was a problem with her bank. The manager had contacted me two weeks prior to my arrival with some concerns. I told her I would be there in two weeks and would drop in to talk to her. Well, as it turned out, Mom had come into the branch on a couple of occasions and wanted to withdraw a large sum of money. Even though they knew her, she was still required to show identification, which she did not have. Her explanation was—you guessed it—"My purse was stolen." Of course, the bank refused to allow her to withdraw money. Keep in mind I was paying all her bills, so there was no reason for her wanting to withdraw a large sum of money. Our concern was maybe she was being scammed—not an uncommon thing to happen to the elderly.

According to the bank manager, Mom tried on another occasion to withdraw a large sum of money, and again she was denied. This time she could not articulate why she needed the money. Her response was *"the man needed it."* She has this thing about *"the man"* with no name. When she is trying to explain something, invariably she uses this phrase as a way of identifying the person of whom she is speaking. I am grateful that Mom had the foresight to add me to her account in 1997.

There were other signs that something was not right with her like she complained that something was wrong with her car or she would forget how to lock the car, forget some routine functions of her car and so on. We would have the car inspected and nothing would be wrong with it. She complained that someone was stealing gas from her car. She especially targeted her next-door neighbor. She felt that he was out to get her. To this day, I am not sure if this was entirely true or not.

My mother has always been meticulous with her hygiene and the clothes she wore. Her clothes now looked dirty. Hygiene-wise she was still bathing but she would put dirty clothes on. She may have forgotten how to use the washer and dryer.

Toward the end of 2018, it was apparent that we could not drag our feet about removing her from the home. Mom was living in a home where the gas in her stove was shut off. Her cooking habits had deteriorated to the point that it became necessary to shut down the stove. She was left with cooking via microwave. As a result, her food consumption suffered.

In October 2018, Zee and I flew home with the express purpose of bringing Mom back with us. We knew it would not be an easy job convincing her to leave, but it was a needful one. When we arrived, Mom had no heat circulating in the house. The house was cold, and she was walking around with a coat on. The pilot light to the furnace had gone out. She did not know how to light it. This, however, was not the first time we encountered her living in a cold house. Zee again had to figure out the problem and fix it. For him it was after a long day of traveling from the west coast to the east coast. I thank God for a good man like my husband. He walks with me every step of the way. He is a blessing to me and our family in so many ways.

Well, by the end of the weekend, we discussed with Mom our plans for bringing her back to California. At first, she tried to convince us to let her remain in the home and she would begin packing things up in preparation to sell her home. Mind you, we had discussed this for the last two years, and yet she had not made any progress to that end. When she realized we were not giving in, she then got angry with us and tried to manipulate us, but we stood firm and would not relent because it was in her best interest that she come with us. Our flight was scheduled to depart at 6:00 a.m. The airport shuttle was picking us up at 3:00 a.m. Right up to midnight, she was adamant about not leaving. I told her we were leaving with or without her. We prefer that she be with us, that it is for her welfare that she goes, and that we love her and need her to allow us to care for her. At this point, I went to bed. Around 1:00 a.m. she came to our room and reluctantly agreed to leave. I packed her bags and off to California we went.

Little did I realize how life changing this decision would be for our family. The adventure of living with someone with dementia cannot adequately be expressed. We are now experiencing the highs, the lows, and the in-betweens of living with dementia daily. I was not prepared for it! All I knew was my mother needed help and it was my duty to help her.

We brought her into our home, thinking we could resume our daily routine with minimal disruption. Au contraire, we work nine-hour days, so we would leave Mom alone in the house. I would come home for lunch to check on her. For a moment, we didn't notice anything different—not until things started going missing. At first, we assumed we misplaced them, but after 3 months, we figured out that Mom was putting things in the trash.

One day, I came home for lunch, opened the garage, and there she was, standing and waving to me. My first thought—she must have locked herself out of the house. Turns out she was going through things in our garage. My husband has tools and fluids for vehicles there. Not a place she should be. The potential for her injuring herself loomed. It had not occurred to me that we must treat her like she was a child. That realization came later.

On a different occasion, I noticed a hole carved out the wall in the garage. She had carved a hole about the size of her fist near the garage door scanner. At this point, we installed a new lock on the garage door.

On three separate times, I came home to a house smelling of gas. She had turned the burner halfway on. Zee had to install in the back of the stove a gas line with a shut-off valve. So when we're away, we shut off the gas.

In our guest bathroom, we had to remove all bathroom cleaners, additional soaps, sanitizers, and medicines. She would put things on her face thinking it was lotion. Twice she sustained burns on her face, so all drawers were emptied as a precaution. She would have liquid soap caked in her scalp. By this time, we began seeking outside help. We hired caregivers to be with her during the day. This has been a tremendous help.

Sometime around March or April 2019, Mom's communication ability declined drastically. She was no longer speaking coherently. There were times when her communication was clear, but those times have become less and less.

We had to consistently navigate her conversation minefields about going home and getting her clothes and seeing about her house. When we resisted, she would get angry and argue with us, accusing me of taking her money and holding her hostage.

My mother has always been adept at articulating herself, so she would get me into a war of words. It frustrated me to no end. The more I tried explaining that she was not well, the more she attacked me. She would approach me with "Can I ask you a question?" More times than not, that was a loaded question because it would lead me down a road of confrontation.

One morning, as I was about to leave for work (before we had a caregiver), she started in about going home and wanting me to give her money. I tried to deflect the conversation, but she was persistent. As I tried to walk away, she blocked me and pushed me up against our 100-gallon fish tank. I pushed her arm up and away. She spun around and fell to the ground. She lay there like she was unconscious. She did not hit her head or anything like that. As she lay there, I told her she must stop this, that I am only trying to help her, that it is my heart for her to be with family in her twilight years, for us to love her and care for her. Then I said, "Ok, let me help you up."

As I tried helping her, she snatched her arm from me and refused to get up from the floor. I said, "Alright, Mom, lay there if you want." I got into my car and called my friend Jackie and asked her to come by and check on Mom. We had cameras installed for monitoring, so I could see if she was still lying on the floor. She was up and about in the house. Jackie came by, but Mom would not answer the door.

Two weeks later, she had a doctor's appointment. At the check-in, I presented Mom's driver's license. The receptionist returned it to me. When we got to the exam room, she started asking me for her driver's license. I did not want her to have it because I knew it would be misplaced and we would need it for other things. After the doctor's exam, she started up again about the license. As I started to stand up, she grabbed my jacket, pulling me back down. I was in a half-standing position, trying to get her to loosen her grip.

It seems they have a supernatural strength when angry. I could hear my jacket about to rip. Her voice was raised, and no doubt, the folks in the front office heard the commotion. I relented and gave her the license. I was very upset with her that day. As predicted, she misplaced the license. I found it a month later.

In November 2019, Mom, her granddaughters, great granddaughter, and I went on a girls' trip to see the *Donna Summer Musical Review* at the Pantages Theater in Los Angeles. We were celebrating my eldest, Carla's birthday. Our day started off great. We had lunch, saw the musical and had dinner. On our way home, things suddenly changed. Mom was sitting in the front passenger seat when she decided to pour water on the console where my phone was sitting. I asked her to stop, and the girls (her granddaughters, Carla and Christine, and great granddaughter, Ebony) tried to clean up the area while I continued driving. At this point, Mom became combative with them and me. I had to pull off the highway and try to get control of the situation.

I asked her to change seats and sit in the second row, but she refused to move. When Carla tried to unbuckle Mom's seat belt, she kicked Carla in the stomach, sending her tumbling backward. Christine attempted to talk Mom down. All the while, Ebony is in the back, crying. Chris was able to coax Mom out of the car. Now we are standing on the side of the highway at ten o'clock at night. Traffic was zooming by us, and the temp was 47 degrees. She is refusing to re-enter the car while telling us the man was talking to her. We were able calm her down and attempted to put her back in the car.

As I was guiding her by her arm, she suddenly jerked her arm from my hand and swirled around with her back to oncoming traffic. She began backing up into approaching traffic. I yelled and grabbed her, snatching her out of harm's way. She then yanked herself away from me and turned and fell on the ground. It looked like she hit her head. She appeared to be unconscious. Carla dialed 911 and I tried to revive her, but she lay motionless.

The fire department and EMTs were dispatched. As I talked with the dispatcher, he asked what happened and to check for bleeding behind her head. I did and there was not. He asked us to check for consciousness but there was no response. We attempted to move her farther away from the highway when she stiffened up. So, she was conscious. He told us to let her lie there but keep her warm. When we saw the emergency lights approaching, we again attempted to get her to sit up. This time she responded.

When the first responders arrived, she acted like nothing happened. In fact, she started flirting with the EMTs. She was smiling and cooperative with them. We all stood back in utter amazement. It was like two different people. They took her vitals, examined her head, talked with her, then put her in the rear seat. What a way to end the day. A day we shall never forget.

In December 2017, Mother was visiting us for the Christmas season. As a surprise, her niece was driving from Arizona to California to visit family. We arranged with Sheila to meet us in San Diego on December 22nd. Sheila was one of her favorite nieces. We arrived at the Naval Station at 32nd St. and checked into the Navy Lodge. Mom had her room and we had ours.

Around midnight, the front desk called our room to inform us that Mom was in the lobby and asked us to come down. Upon arrival, the front desk clerk informed us that Mom had approached her, requesting a cab to take her back to Philadelphia. This same clerk had checked us in and noticed some behaviors Mom was displaying during our check-in. I explained to the clerk that Mom was suffering from dementia, and she understood because she is dealing with it with her in-laws. I am grateful to her for taking a proactive posture with Mom and notifying us.

We escorted Mom back to her room and tried to explain why we were in San Diego. She, at this point, would not be appeased. She claimed we had kidnapped her and on and on... Zee tried to reason with her but to no avail, so we told her the reason for the trip—it was to be a surprise for her seeing her niece—but even that bit of news did not affect her. She was adamant in her position, and of course, we all were wrong.

On Sheila's arrival the next day, Mom acted as if nothing from the previous night happened—because in her mind, nothing did. We had a lovely visit after starting off rough.

April 2021: A normal day until the afternoon, when Mom decided to leave our caregiver's home and take a stroll through the neighborhoods. Mind you, my mother has always been a fast walker, and once she got out of the front door, she was off to the races. Before Jackie knew it, Mom had crossed a busy intersection and was about to enter someone's home. The homeowners had left their home unlocked and Mom walked right in. She then locked the door and Jackie ran up to the house, knocking on the door, asking Mom to unlock the door. She eventually did.

Jackie was escorting her off the property when a neighbor drove up and asked if everything was alright. Jackie explained that Mom had dementia and she was trying to get her back home. The neighbor came up to Mom, trying to assist Jackie with her. Mom then turned around and punched him in the face. They were able to get her into the car, but she was refusing to put her legs in. While they were attempting to put her legs in, she would begin hitting the person.

I was headed home from work when I got the call from Jackie about the situation. Zee and I arrived at the same time. We tried talking to her, trying to convince her to allow us to put her legs into the car, but to no avail, so we forced the issue. We put her in and secured the seat belt on her and I sat in the back with her while Victor, Jackie's husband, drove my car home. On the way, Mom kept punching and biting me until I asked Jackie to pull over. Zee got in the back on the other side of Mom to hold her hands. For a little lady of approximately 100 lbs., she had the strength of two people.

At this juncture, emotionally I had reached my limit. I knew we as a family could not continue this way. Mom needed to be in a facility that could provide the needed services for her. Our home—our family—was not equipped to continue with the daily care for Mom.

So, the next day began my search for a place for Mom. Through God's providence, we were connected to a facility. Arrangements were made, and we moved Mom to her new and current and final location. The facility is seventy miles south of us. We see her often.

Her adjustment to her new home was not a smooth one. She was combative and refused to comply. They resorted to giving her anti-anxiety medications which calmed her down considerably. At the time of this writing, Mom had been at the facility for seventeen months. She has adjusted to her new surroundings.

This is an abbreviated history of what Mom and our family have gone through. I did not speak about the countless times of her speaking harshly to her great grands and not wanting to be near them or her hiding her meds, telling me she has taken them or the times she would just take a swing at me, etc. The whole ordeal was physically and emotionally exhausting, but I kept remembering God's Word: *"Children, honor your father and mother so that it may be well with you."*

We have many stories that my children tell and laugh about. We love her dearly and are sorry for what dementia has done to her. Dementia has robbed us of precious moments with her, but before dementia, we have a treasure trove of memories that we will cherish.

As you read my stories, understand this is a snapshot and a glimpse into what families currently are dealing with regarding dementia and the care of their loved ones. It is no small task!

Countless families are dealing with loved ones suffering from dementia. Dear friends of ours tell us about a time when the wife's mother was lost in the desert. They awoke one morning to find her gone. They searched for her for almost a day before she was found. She was unharmed when found.

A friend spoke of her mother's anger over receiving help from her family. All she wanted to do was to sit at home and drink alcoholic beverages during the day. She got to the point where her anger became unbearable for the family to handle, so they put her in a facility. Doing that caused her to accuse her children of not caring for her. She remained very angry until the day she passed away. The situation was very disheartening to this family because all their efforts were centered from caring, loving hearts. They wanted to do what's best for her, but she made it difficult for every family member.

One day I received a knock at the door. There stood a police officer. Apparently, dispatch received a 911 call from my home. It was mother calling and telling dispatch that she was a prisoner. Of course, they must check out the call. I reassured them all is well with Mom, that she has dementia. They looked around and talked with Mom, but she did not tell them what she reported to dispatch. In fact, she acted like nothing was wrong.

Who can speak of the countless discoveries of medicines, food, knives, eyeglasses, and small portable things found in her room, under her mattress, in the closet, things hidden in her purses or hidden in clothes—it required frequent assessments of her room—or the dismantling of lamps, the tearing pages out of books, or things missing, never to be found.

The Bible says that a king should never go to war before first counting the cost.

For which of you, wishing to build a farm building, does not first sit down and calculate the cost [to see] whether he has sufficient means to finish it?

Otherwise, when he has laid the foundation and is unable to complete [the building], all who see it will begin to mock {and} jeer at him,

Saying, this man began to build and was not able (worth enough) to finish.

Or what king, going out to engage in conflict with another king, will not first sit down and consider {and} take counsel whether he is able with ten thousand [men] to meet him who comes against him with twenty thousand?

And if he cannot [do so], when the other king is still a great way off, he sends an envoy and asks for the terms of peace. Luke 14:28-32 *amplified*

Well, that same premise applies when faced with a monumental decision to care for a loved one with dementia. Our way of life would be drastically altered. The engineering changes required for our household were not a consideration. Changing locks throughout the home, adding cameras, removing household items from cabinets, and emotionally staying alert for any possibility was not factored in. Essentially one must *Mom-proof* their home like one does for a baby. One must screen what is eaten too. In a sense, there is a reverting back to infancy-like behavior. This was something we were not prepared for.

We certainly did not count the cost prior to bringing Mother into our home. Our primary thought was rescuing Mom from her current situation and providing the security, stability and care she needed. How that would be achieved would be answered later—and later came fast!

Our story is not unique to us; rather, it is the norm today. More and more families are facing the dilemma of what to do for loved ones with dementia.

I don't have the answers, but I can testify to what we have walked through as a family. I can say this—you don't have to go through this alone. Search out organizations, groups, and people who can give advice and comfort to you during these challenging times.

In the next chapter, I will talk about what helped us navigate life with Mom.

I hope we shared a smile, laugh or giggle about some of the funny things we encountered on this journey with Mom.

CHAPTER 4

Help!

"My grace is sufficient for you.
For My strength is made perfect in weakness."
1 Corinthians 12:9

When we started this journey with Mom, we consulted a few organizations regarding her physical state. We had a reasonable idea of what to expect in the days and years to come, but we did not know how to correctly respond to situations with Mom—for instance, the constant accusations of us/me stealing her money or claims we are holding her against her will, etc.

As mentioned in earlier chapters, Mom was very skillful with words. She was masterful in getting one frustrated during conversation—and forget about trying to correct her assertions; they fell on deaf ears.

For me, the most perplexing thing was how could she think so badly of me or the family when all we wanted to do was help her navigate and mitigate what she was going through. Sadly, she did not see it that way, so you can imagine how frustrated we became facing the daily verbal accusations and at times followed with her physically lashing out at us. For a moment, I felt like I was living in a war zone, not knowing where or when the attacks would come from—because one moment things would be fine and the next moment some other person would emerge with anger and indifference. That was baffling to all of us, especially to her great grandchildren. They would ask me, "What is wrong with Great Grandmom? Why did she say this or that?"

We would explain that Great Grandmom was ill, and she did not mean what she said or did. Our explanations helped ease some of their fears, and their fears were legitimate because Mom continued demonstrating erratic behavior, but to a five-year-old who just wanted to be near and around her was a tall order. Complicating matters, Mom would encourage her grandkids to come and talk to her, and the next day she didn't want anything to do with them. I knew we had to do something to change the atmosphere at home.

One day at work, I spoke about Mom's status to a co-worker, who suggested that I consult Senior Services. I contacted them and discovered a caregiver support group for those caring for family members. The first night I attended was so refreshing and encouraging to me. Discovering that I was not alone was huge. I heard testimony after testimony of varying family situations and dynamics of caregivers trying to help their loved ones.

One such lady was a caregiver to both mom and dad. She expressed how little personal time she had. Most of her day was devoted to the care of her parents. The support group was her only outlet, and how she relished her times away. I thoroughly identified with her. Her mother had physical limitations while her dad was dealing with dementia. My heart went out to her. My family dynamics were different in that I had my family assisting, especially when things got hairy with Mom. I could break away for some personal time.

One person spoke about the limited services in our town and the frustration over not having adequate assistance. Small towns suffer from a lack of needed services for families, so families are left to handle and manage on their own. Thank God for friends and a church family that was willing to step in and help—but not everyone has that to rely upon.

My breakthrough came from one of those evening sessions. The facilitator's name was Daryl. He went around the room, asking how our week had gone. I had experienced an intensely trying week with Mom. I reiterated what transpired and when finished, Daryl said to me, *"Connie, you cannot let your mother pull you into her world. The more she does it, it is frustrating to you because she will have you spun up over things. She is not conscious of what she's doing or saying.* **All she knows is her world is upside down and she is frustrated with not knowing what's happening to her.** *Step out of her world. Recognize that you are her caregiver now. You must learn to divorce yourself from being her daughter. You are her caregiver now."*

Boy, was that liberating to me and at the same time challenging. I was raised with a healthy respect for authority. I especially honor our seniors. It was so hard for me to look at Mom not as Mom, but in the long run, Daryl's words would reverberate within me time and time again as I navigated stormy moments with Mom. *Connie, you are a caregiver to Mom.*

Daryl also encouraged us to get out and away from the situation as much as we could and for us to continue living our lives as much as possible while knowing the situation may get worse as the dementia progresses. Reality check—the Mother I knew was not coming back unless God intervened, which was my prayer. All my dreams of Mom and I traveling after I retired were flushed down the drain. My dreams of her and I catching up on missed times together would not materialize. These things I had to settle in my heart. That was a struggle that even to this day I am not completely over with.

So, what does one do in these types of situations? Well, you seek out family first for their assistance. In some family situations, family members live in other states or far away from the person or persons needing care. If you are the one caring for someone, then seek out professional help and community organizations for assistance. Every community typically maintains a list of available services. You may not need everything that is offered but avail yourself and your loved one to as much as possible.

- Some services that may be available are:
- Transportation referrals
- Meals on Wheels referrals
- Information regarding caregiver support groups
- Alzheimer's disease information, including applications for respite grants
- Assistance completing basic forms
- Transitional Care
- Personal Care
- Pharmacy

Case Management: Provides the above services for an individual who may need extra assistance. These folks require short-term assistance, either on a weekly or monthly basis.

Homemakers Program: Provides non-medical housekeeping services in the home. Examples are light housekeeping, laundry, meal prep, grocery shopping, and socialization. Most people receive services every other week for two hours.

These are my local services. Seek out churches in your area for any family-related services. Don't try and do this alone. We all need assistance, whether we're giving the care or the one receiving the care. With more and more families facing the possibility of caring for a loved one, it is so important that you ask for help. There is help.

If you are faced with caring long term for a loved one with dementia or a physical malady, obtaining a power of attorney is vital! I cannot underscore the necessity of this legal document. It helps tremendously in transacting business on their behalf.

The rise of dementia presents a unique challenge to the family—particularly if the family member is physically fine and the only major problem is dementia. Dementia presents its own set of unique problems. It is an emotionally draining experience for caregivers, family, and the person affected. Seek out help.

CHAPTER 5

Going Home

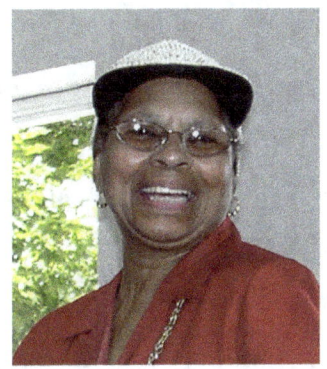

I once was told by a dear friend, Jennifer Silberberg, that dementia is a slow walk home. How right she was. I began writing this book in 2020. At the time of completion, 2024, Mom had already gone home to be with the Lord in January 2023.

I received a call from her nurse on Monday, January 02, 2023. I was told that she had stopped eating the day before. I went to see her on Tuesday, January 3rd. When I saw her, she looked very different. I remember Mother telling me how people looked when death is imminent. I remember feeling the rush of feelings flood my soul and much regret for not having more time with her. At this point, she was barely conscious. I sat and read scripture to her and prayed over her. I told her how much I loved her and so on. This was not the time to hold anything back. I needed her to know that despite the fact we had no father in our lives, she was a wonderful mother. She made up for what we lacked in not having one, that if Keith and I could have chosen our mother, she would be the one we chose.

I called Keith and put him on speaker, and he too said basically the same things I said to her. He prayed over her as well. I then called her sister, Iona, and she talked to Mom about their times growing up. It was a sweet and precious time. I returned home later that evening.

On Thursday, January 5th, I returned and spent the better part of the day with her. This time, her eyes were open, and she appeared to be more in the moment than on my previous visit. She was laboring a bit in her breathing but appeared to be calm and looking around and looking at me. By this time, she had lost the ability to speak. Again, I called Keith and he talked to her, and we both read scripture to her. I could sense a presence in the room with us. I have read accounts regarding believers and their transitioning time from this earth to heaven, how angels are present to escort them into the presence of the living God.

I sensed we needed to release her from this life to be with the Lord—this I said to Keith—and so, he began the process of releasing Mom. He told her how wonderful of a mother she had been to us, that we couldn't have a better mom! That we, her family, especially he and I, would be alright, that she had done a good job in raising us, that we would look out for one another just like she taught us to! That it is alright for her to go.

At that moment, a tear dropped from her eyes. We knew she heard us! When the call ended, I called Aunt Iona.

Aunt Iona talked with her again about their childhood and all the good times they had and how blessed she was to have a sister like her. She too released Mom. She told Mom it was okay for her to go and that she loved her. Again, a tear came down Mom's face. Once she concluded her call, then it was my turn. Boy, I did not want to release her. I wanted her to stay here with me as long as she could, but I know that was selfish of me—but she's my mommy, and I did not want to see her go. And yet I know from scripture that we shall see her again.

"I am the resurrection and the life. He who believes in Me, though he may die, he shall live." John 11:25

So I began telling her how blessed our family is because of her. I thanked her for all the sacrifices she made for Keith and me. I told her again what a wonderful job she did in raising us. In years gone by, Mom had expressed a regret in working too much and not spending more time with us. We understood she had to do what she had to do. On her off days, she spent them with us doing family things. She kept us in church and was always present in our lives as a parent. There was no doubt in our minds that Mom loved us! I did not want her entering eternity thinking otherwise. I expressed how much I loved her and how much I will miss her! I prayed scripture over her then I released her.

I said, *"Mom, it's ok. You can go home now. Keith and I will be fine. You have instilled in us valuable qualities that will live on in us and in our children. We will look out for one another just like you taught us to. It's ok, Mom, I release you!"* And again, for the third time, a tear dropped from her eyes.

I departed for home shortly afterwards. In the early hours of the following morning, around 1:35 a.m., I received a call from her nurse informing me that she had passed.

I am so grateful to my heavenly Father for giving us the opportunity to say our goodbyes and share our hearts with her this side of heaven.

Since her passing, my family have laughed at the many hilarious moments with Mom. She lives on in our hearts and memories. We know we shall see her again! We are blessed to be a part of her life. We have since heard countless stories of how our mother was a friend to many, how she gave to others and how she loved serving others.

Lillian Williams has left us a legacy to follow—a legacy of love, faithfulness, commitment, joy, and family. Mother taught us that no matter what the problem or situation, one could always get a chuckle from it. Mother loved to laugh. In fact, her siblings laughed often when they were together—a legacy she has passed on to us and our children and our children's children.

As the scripture says, *"A merry heart does good like medicine."*

So, to those reading this book, despite the trials and challenges you may face, find joy in the laughter and cherish the moments. Might as well laugh!

Thank you for allowing me to share our family story of our beloved mother, Lillian Williams.

May the words of this book bless you!

NOTES

1. WebMD LLC 2020
2. Caroline Leaf, MD, *Who Switched Off My Brain?*
3. New Spirit Filled Life Bible, Thomas Nelson Publishers, Nashville, TN. 1982
4. Dr. Barry Reisberg, Director of Fisher Alzheimer's Disease Education and Research, NYU Grossman School of Medicine.
5. www.alzinfo.org